Happiness & Lollipops

A difficult journey in a difficult mind

Foreword:

To everyone involved in my life thank you. Your constant support is touching and I love you all. My road has been a rocky one but with you by my side it makes that road just a little bit smoother.

Chapter One: Another Introduction

I fucking irritate myself, I truly mean that. I wish that I had an identity, a persona. Instead I adapt myself to the people around me, I'm a social chameleon and I don't fucking like it. I'm too scared to be myself around people, I'm too worried that I won't be everyone's friend and I'm scared that I say something that won't be in line with the company I find myself in at any particular time. I'm 33 and I'm still trying to find myself, I don't know what I think of myself and I just cannot seem to get going at all.

So what's been happening since I last wrote, I now have no job, I'm back living with my parents as I have no flat and oh yea', I nearly committed suicide back in December, so yea', nothing has happened at all.... I am so fucking sick of my head, I'm hateful of the person I am and I'm hateful of my uncanny ability to not know what the fuck is going on inside of me. I don't think I'll ever be faulted on effort, I put so much in each and every single day and although things have been good lately a lot of that has been down to me and turning negatives into positives. Do you know something I'll say this before I start getting into this and it's the one thing I feel I know about myself: I HATE society and I hate being forced to be a part of their fads, trends and fucking obsessions with music. I drink a lot but when I do it helps me to escape the mind-numbing humdrum of the daily grind. On reflection I think it would be better if I were to be cast adrift from society and left to drive myself insane.

So it's been over three months since I wrote all of the above and I'm pleased to report that I am in a much better, stronger place now, at the time of writing that I was in such a bad place and to be honest I think I was a little bit raw from my attempted suicide on 28/12/2014. So before I start delving into things I'm going to go through a couple of things that's happened. At the time of writing it's 24/05/2015 and it's bang on 11am. Lots has happened since I last wrote and the majority has been great. So what's been happening in my life, well instead of being called Dave I've decided to take my father's name so I am now called Davy, I've managed to secure a really good job and I've decided to devote my life to being completely and utterly celibate, so yea', both me and my mind have been busy.

I think I'll start with the celibacy thing, it just feels like the right place to begin things, it's the biggest decision I've made in my life up until this point and I'll explain the reasoning why, I didn't really touch on it in my previous book but then again at the time of my previous writings I really wasn't in a great place at all, infact who I am I kidding at the time of writing my last one I was close to death, I did state at the end I may not make it through this and at the end of December I tried to quit, I overdosed and I had made my peace with it. I had said my goodbyes and that was it. I took about 30 tablets, I can't remember the exact name of them but I remember the feeling of my chest tightening up almost immediately and me sitting on my bed ready to die. I text my brother saying goodbye and that I was sorry for putting him through this but enough was enough. The previous week I stood on the balcony of my top floor flat and nearly jumped, I was hospitalised twice in a week. I really came **THAT** close, I mean I actually attempted to take my own life, actually just writing this and thinking about it I 'm really grateful to all around me, I have an amazing support network and they got me through a phenomenally horrible time. Infact it wasn't just horrible for me it was horrible for everyone concerned. I never ever want to put my family through that again. I will never ever forget the look on their faces when I came to in hospital.

So over the last five months I've been solely focused on building my mental strength, it's been a long road but I finally feel strong within myself again, I feel like I've always felt I should be. I feel confident, I feel strong and I feel ready to kick on. I'll be 100% honest, I genuinely don't think I give myself nearly enough credit for the amount of strength I have and the things I have actually achieved, I am way too harsh on myself and that's one of the many things that I have actually managed to banish. As this goes on and I start to delve deep inside me I'll try to take you with me and try to let you see what I see and feel what I feel. I'll try, I can't make any guarantees you'll see it but I'll do my absolute best. At points as well I'll be writing after having a few beers, with just the right amount it helps me open up a little bit more, I'll let you know when that happens as well, throughout this I will hopefully be able to fully delve and come out of this even stronger.

Make no mistakes this is going to be hard for me. Everything that I write is going to present it's own obstacle or challenge. I don't want you thinking that me writing this is going to be a cakewalk. This is going to be fucking hard work because what I'm going to do is basically strip myself down, break myself open, expose myself at my weakest and then look to build myself back up, now that's territory I've been to before but not to the extent that I'm going to attempt in writing this book. The first one compared to this was easy because I was at my absolute lowest, the words came easy as the feelings were at my fingertips, this I think is going to be a lot tougher to write.

Chapter Two: Wiring

I'm not saying this just to be different and I'm certainly not saying it to make myself sound cool, I'm saying this because I genuinely believe it. My wiring is different to the majority of society's, it's something that I've always believed and I do think I feel more than the average person. I have a tremendous amount of empathy, it's at a point where I use it almost for 95% of conversations, I can't help it, when someone is speaking I almost always jump into an empathetic state of mind, it happens automatically like just getting up and washing my face or putting my pants and socks on at the start of my day, I mean it just happens. Now that doesn't sound normal to me, it's something that has always happened and I can't turn it off. I'm not saying it's a bad thing, I'm just saying I think it's different and it allows me straight away to 'feel' my way around a conversation more than an average person. I'd like to point out straight away I'm not saying I have a totally unique mindset, I'm trying to point out a number of different factors that all contribute to my struggles and battles with depression.

I am way too much of a nice guy, I'm nice to the point where sometimes I actually want to punch myself in the face, yea' it sounds harsh but it's true, I bend over backwards for people and I always put other's needs before my own. Once again it's something I've always done.

I over-think, I mean I really over-think, my head never switches off and this is something I touched on in great detail in my previous work. I don't think this helps, I really don't.. I would love nothing more than for my brain to switch off but I just don't have that capability. Plus a lot of the time I never really know what's going on inside my head and by that I mean I'm always unsure of what other people's perceptions are of me, this is a **HUGE** factor in my depressive state, this is the one thing that cripples me when I have my bad days and the reason for that is that this one thought, this one conundrum in my mind wears me down and I never stop thinking about it. I mean this is an actual obsession, touch wood that it's not been bad lately but when it strikes it causes me to (over) analyse every single thing I do. Some typical examples of this are:

- Speaking:

    - Hmm, could I have made that better?
    - Was my tone inflection correct?
    - Was my emphasis right?
    - Oh fuck did they think I was a cheeky fucker there, oh shit..
    - Why did I say that, she hates me now.
    - Fuck you Davy, you've blew it.

- General:

    - Am I walking ok?
    - Do I look confident?
    - Don't look down. Don't look down, you **need** to look confident
    - Your music is too loud
    - Do the people on the train think this band is ok?
    - Am I dressed ok today? What if I'm not dressed well.

I mean I don't know if any of that makes sense but that's a little bit of what I go through when I'm having a not so good day, I refuse to say bad day now because that just amplifies/increases the speed of my thoughts. I've learned a lot from my depression and I think I'm managing it better. On 97% of my days these thoughts don't even enter my head, I'm confident, personable, attentive and ready to attack whatever the day has in-store for me, but on the 'not so good days' it's an achievement I'm actually able to get out of my bed and believe me, that is hard work on one of those days. It.. is... fucking.... awful.. *sad face*

I don't know why I care so much about people's perceptions of me. I mean at the end of the day does it really matter? I mean really, DOES IT MATTER? The honest and direct answer is no, it really fucking doesn't. (You'll see my language really hasn't improved at all throughout this, honestly it's fine though, I think it makes it easier to get points across. I may be wrong but I can't be the judge of that. The truth is I like swearing, end of)

All of the above (with the exception of swearing) I have really put a lot of effort into and I think now I've managed to eradicate a lot of the self-doubt and the panicking. It's still a work in progress but I think I'm doing ok. Infact no scrap that, I don't 'think I'm doing ok', I AM doing ok. No actually I'm doing well. I need to be more positive, I've been working on being more positive and it's definitely making a difference, plus for the first time in years I'm actually comfortable in my own skin, that makes a massive difference both psychologically and socially. I think this is the strongest

I've ever felt, I actually feel really good within myself and that comes across. I'm not doubting myself as much, I'm not over-thinking as much and I think I am looking really good. I think I decided to practice celibacy at the wrong time. D'oh!

That leads me on to another point. A lot of the time in my head things have always been 'wrong', whether they actually were wrong or if it was just a state of mind have yet to be proven, I contributed a lot to my own problems because I didn't manage my state of mind correctly. For example on a particularly stressful day at work I would deal with this by 'having a few drinks', now my definition of a few drinks differs. When I'm out with friends me going for a few drinks generally involves a night out, the standard term is to go out and have 'a few drinks', when I'd had a not so good day a few drinks meant I would go to the shop, buy six cans of beer, have them and do that over three to four days a week, so I wasn't just having a few beers, I had an alcohol problem and I was using a bad day as an excuse to drink, there is a massive difference between the two and to be honest I lead myself to drink a lot of the 'bad/not so good days'. I've always had a dependency on alcohol, at my worst it's really quite bad though.

It's hard a lot of the time, I mean it really is, from the time I left 3 on 02/05/2014 and by the time I went off sick from my last employer so much had changed within me, I wasn't the same person and I think a lot of it was to do with the fact that I didn't have that 'support network' in a professional environment, before I could go into work, have a quiet day and not talk to anyone and it went from that to going in every day and hiding how I was feeling. People at 3 understood me and they knew I would have a couple of days downtime then be back to my usual self again. In my last job I didn't have that and I made the cataclysmic mistake of hiding my depression, the end result being on 01/09/2014 I lost control, I couldn't hide it anymore and I broke down, that was the start of the worst ever period of my life and if I could do the whole thing again I would do it so much different. Actually, one thing that definitely didn't help was the fact that I pissed away a sizeable redundancy in the space of three months. I would tell you just how much I pissed away but you'd never look at me the same again.

Just before I continue here's a quick question. What do you think I blew my redundancy on? Was it:

a) A holiday
b) Strippers
c) Booze

Yip you're right, I did manage to blow a lot of my money on nights out because I was 'happy', yea' I wasn't happy, I was an alcoholic with basically a large amount of tokens, looking back on it I did not handle the transition well. Thankfully though I am now in a place where I can look at it, acknowledge it and move on whereas before I would look at it, analyse it, over-analyse it, think about it, agonize about it and then worry about it. Having a much sharper, clearer state of mind helps me to review things rather than over-analyse things, generally as well I am now looking forward rather than living in my past, it helps, believe me.

Even though that happened a while ago it still hurts a lot, at the start of this remember I said this wasn't going to be easy for me? Yea' that stings a bit going back over it and not just for what I've written. See I was off from the start of September and I didn't handle my time off well either. Although I had a really fragile state of mind I don't think I approached it the right way. See the problem I had was that I was alone a lot and the reason for that was because some days I just couldn't face anyone, now that in itself was fine but I spent a lot of my days just wandering around the house in my pyjamas and then just playing xBox, I didn't really adventure out, I shut the curtains and I basically barricaded myself inside my house, I also didn't wash my face for about three months, infact I didn't wash my face from 01/09/2014 until 24/11/2014.

Now under normal circumstances I would be thinking the same as you, I'd be like 'eww, three months without washing your face, gros'. Yea' it would have been but when you suffer you don't see it like that. What did I have to wash my face for? I wasn't seeing anyone, I wasn't doing anything. All I would do is get up in the morning, have breakfast and then put the xBox on, that is all that I would do and that went on for months. I wandered from room-to-room thinking what am I doing, I found it hard to see my parents because I couldn't let them know how I was feeling, I struggled to talk to my friends, I couldn't. What would I say? I didn't know what to say to them. I didn't even know what was going on in my own head for fuck sake. It took all my effort to get up and out of bed, that in itself was a huge achievement, some days I would even open the curtains but that was on a REALLY good day, I mean that was on a REALLY GOOD DAY, they didn't come along often though. Looking back on it I actually spent a lot of time living like a recluse, I didn't particularly enjoy it but well, it happened and I can't really change it.

See this is what makes it hard for me to talk to anyone when I don't feel right within myself, I can convey this all to you and to be honest I don't know what you're thinking, I doubt I'll ever know what you're thinking. All I want to get across really is the fact that as long as I live I will always be battling this. I am always going to be trying to conquer this and I'm accepting that this is my life. I don't think that I would want it any other way to be honest and I'm going to explain why I wouldn't want to be like anyone else:

I find a lot of life boring, this socialistic ideal of the wife and two kids by the time you're in your thirties just pisses me off. Getting the nice suburban house that everyone else in your street has just doesn't appeal to me. Doing the garden on your day off and taking the kids to the park just doesn't cut it for me and besides, I've got more than enough to manage on my own never mind if you throw in a wedding, a wife and the thought of me being a father, that just flat terrifies me. I'm quite happy being on my own but then I know if I'm on my own I can make my own timetable, obviously now I'm back in work I'm referring to managing my time out of work. How would I manage my mental state with having a wife and kids, how would I get across to them that I needed some time on my own, what would I do if I got one of THOSE days where I physically couldn't talk to anyone? One of those days where I have to be on my own and there's nothing I could do? One of THOSE days where I end up wandering around Falkirk or Glasgow aimlessly with the simple intention of just... killing time? I don't think I could do it, would the wife understand? What about the kids? How would I explain that 'Dad just needs some time on his own', this can happen for days at a time, this doesn't limit itself to one day, I mean could I do that? I don't see myself being able to manage that.

And this brings me back to the point I made at the start of this chapter, it's all about wiring, we're all wired different but we share some of the same components, I think I share a lot of the same wiring but there's just that odd switch or two that causes my thinking and my being to be a little deeper than your average joe. Then again though are my thoughts and my fears different than anyone else's? Is it maybe just all in my head and I am actually normal? I just perceive myself to be different in the hope it distinguishes me just that little bit from everyone else? Or am I actually different in terms of the waves of thoughts that overcome me and threaten to drown me from time-to-time. I genuinely don't know, if I did I probably wouldn't be taking this on and I would probably be doing a regular Sunday job like mowing the garden or painting the fence. There has to be something in the way I feel, I mean there just has to be.

I don't think the things I experience/have experienced are normal. I've managed this(poorly at times) for over fifteen years now, something happened when I was eighteen that triggered this and I don't know what. I mean around that time I first started listening to a lot of Nirvana rather than the mainstream pop that I'd grew up with. Did I maybe hear a lyric that started me thinking, was there something in me that changed? Did I have a chemical imbalance that peaked that year, I don't know regrettably but I'd love to go back and see what I was like back then. Infact that's something I think about a lot, going back to the year 2000 and living through that year to see what kind of things I was thinking and doing. Did something happen that's been hidden away in the back of my memory or could it be there is just no explanation, maybe it just.. happened and I didn't realise it. All I know is I'll never find out unless I happen to invent something that allows me to go back and honestly would I do it if I had the chance? No, I probably wouldn't because I would most likely fuck myself up, that would be weird going back and being inside your own head all those years ago. Yea', I think it's best if that's just left in the past.

Maybe I'm looking at this in too complex a fashion, maybe there's a way to just simplify all that's in my head rather than getting the world's biggest blackboard and psycho-analyse every single thought that goes through my head. Like rather than me over-thinking and stressing why could I not just let what's happened live in the past and just look to my future. I mean that's what I have been doing since February and the results are pretty good. I think it's a good thing to acknowledge your past but it's definitely not good to try to live in it, I mean that just screws with your head, it certainly did with mines anyways.

I think about death a lot, once again it's just one of those things that's always been there. I don't think of it in terms of like 'I want to die' but I often wonder what actually happens when death comes. I mean do you get the white light and the big flashback, do you get to look down on people and continue to look over your loved ones after you're gone or do you get to come back and do some really cool haunting. I would LOVE to do that, people that I didn't like and I would just fuck with their chi, like when they're in a bath and I would flicker the light, or put some random bread in their toaster. OR I would just move all of their stuff about and drive them nuts. I totally want to be a ghost when I die, I wouldn't be like your stereotypical ghost, I'd be a 'cerebrally talented' ghost, I would so fuck with your head.

But on a serious note what happens when you die, I mean it's one of those things that's really down to your own interpretation I guess, now I'm not going to get into religious beliefs here because quite frankly I often find these discussions/debates rather tedious. I've just often wondered what happens after you go, it's just one of those things that runs round my head.

Chapter Three: Relationships/Celibacy and stuff....

Ugh, I dreaded this bit but if I get it out now then I won't need to cover it later.

I've never really been in a meaningful relationship, the previous partners I've had have all been ok but I don't think I've ever felt the whole love thing. Since the age of eighteen I've had maybe three/four girlfriends and to be honest it's just never really worked. I mean I know a lot of pretty girls, I'm definitely lucky that way and yea' I fancy a few of them but I know in my heart of hearts me and relationships would never really work.

- I lack confidence
- My mental state

That's pretty much it, I mean the relationships I've been in have all broken down because of me, I either just lost interest and in one I actually cheated on my partner, I'm not proud of that. I think I'm just one of those guys who is going to be better off on his own, that was the main reason for my decision a few weeks ago to practice celibacy, the last time I had sex was January 2013 and to be honest I don't miss it. I mean yea' it's nice and if you get the right partner it can be great but I'm not really bothered. I mean I'm really not. I don't have the confidence or the desire needed for a relationship. By deciding to become celibate I've taken a lot of the pressure off of me because I am no longer dressing or acting to try to attract members of the opposite sex, that was one of the big worries in my mind, because I'm naturally insecure I would spend ages in the morning trying on lots of different combinations and instead of picking something I was comfortable in I was picking clothing to try to make myself more appealing to the females I worked/commuted with.

Now, I don't think I'm a bad looking guy, don't get me wrong I'm never going to win Mr Universe or appear in a 'Greatest Hunks of All Time' calendar but I have a lot going for me. I'm not going to list what I feel are my strengths because frankly I've a lot but 99% of the time

I look nice and I smell nice. I wear decent clothing and generally I feel great. The problem I had was that I was trying to attract just anyone, I get attracted to girls quite easy and to all different shapes and sizes, personally I prefer curves but that's my own personal preference. The problem I had was when I first met a girl whether it was in work or on a night out my first thought (if I was attracted to them) was 'Hmm, I wonder if they're single', now that I know for a fact is the complete wrong way to look at someone because 90% of time I'm going to be disappointed as I know they've got a partner, the other 10% would be me just thinking to myself 'Should I ask them out' or 'I wonder if they like me'. Now when I look back on that I realise my mistake and I now no longer do that. When I first meet someone now I just act like myself, also now that I'm not looking for anyone I know that takes a lot of the pressure off because I am comfortable in my own skin and not trying so hard to impress. Women can tell when you're doing that, women know a lot.

At the same time though I mean I don't think I've ever really been that bothered though, I mean yea' there were times when I was looking for a relationship but I was always 'just looking', I never really went out on a lot of dates, I guess that's just the way it happened. To be honest there's too much in my mind I've got to control, that's why I think it's always been best that I'm single and besides, for the first time in a long while I'm now in a place where I am truly happy within myself, if I was to look at being with someone, now would be the time to start looking. I mean I still look at women in a normal way, I still get attracted to them and I still think normally, my celibacy hasn't changed the way I look at them. I'm at a point in my life where I want to start achieving and the new job that I started on 05/05/2015 is definitely the place where I want to be. I need to start looking at goals I want to set, although I'm only thirty-three I'm at a point in my life and my career to really start doing something wonderful. The key thing for me is going to be keeping on top of my mind and ensuring that if there is something wrong I speak to someone about it. I know exactly who to speak to as well should something go wrong.

The relationships I truly treasure are my family and friends, I have had and am still having the privilege of meeting some truly fantastic people, now I only started my new job three weeks ago and I went out on Friday with them and we got absolutely steamin' drunk, I mean we got absolutely shit-faced and legless and this is only after three weeks. I am really lucky in the fact that whatever job I am in I always get a really good training group that I always end up making great friends with, it's the same in any job that I've had I always end up meeting great people and they all mean the world to me. I don't know how I always end up with this happening but I don't care, I hope to know these people for the rest of my life, although I have my struggles and my ups/downs I know these people are going to be there for me, that in itself gives me a lot of strength, I value friendship higher than I value anything else. I could never be one of those people with lots of money with hundreds upon thousands of fake friends. I would rather live my life and have the people I have over thousands of hangers-on who only hang around with me for money. Incidentally, to any of my friends reading this if you are hanging around with me for money I'm afraid I don't have much, sorry! (Laugh out loud) In all seriousness I depend on my friends and family as without them I'm nothing. Without them I have nothing to strive for, nothing to better myself for, I don't have any reason to make myself live for without them. Because I do have them though I can get up in the morning and know I've got to give whatever I do 100%, whether that be the current training I'm doing for my new job, whether it be playing snooker or whether it be going on a night out with the various social circles I have. One thing is for certain, they will always continue to motivate me to be better so to all of you guys I'm lucky to know, thank you from the bottom of my heart. You mean so much to me and you continue to give me strength.

See that to me means one million times more to me than being in a relationship. I don't care much for them but I will always care for my friends. I know that they're always there for me and I'm always there for them. Friendship means more to me than anything and I wouldn't trade the people I had for all the money in the world. That's what made the period from September 2014 until December 2014 the worst of my life, I couldn't see them, I couldn't be with them and most importantly I couldn't talk to them, I couldn't talk to anyone for four months and it almost ended up with me losing my life, I can't even say that I'm sorry because the reasons for dying outweighed the reasons I wanted to live. It was a bloody, mentally draining battle that I fought so hard and so long for and it had won. That's the thing with depression, that's what people can't see, it's a war within the mind and although on the outside I looked fine, internally I was anything but. At the time of writing six months ago I thought I was coming out of it, I genuinely felt that I was making really good progress and in a month or so I'd be back to work, as it turned out I had absolutely no idea just what was going to transpire over the next six to eight weeks.

I use social media a lot, well I use Facebook a lot, I used that as a means to update people around me how things were progressing and I think I used it quite well. It is oh so easy though to lie though, not just on social media but by texting as well. It's easy to stick a smiley face on the end of a post or a message and people can think 'oh he's fine, look he's smiling'. The truth is though that it's dead easy to do that and to fool people, if I could live that period of my life again I would do things differently. I didn't want people worrying, I felt as if my illness was taking up their time, I felt guilty, I felt as if I should just deal with this myself, other people have their own worries you know Davy.

Infact, Davy... why are you doing this? Deal with this yourself because people have stuff going on too. Davy, ok? You deal with this, this is your responsibility, no-one elses.. ok?'

That's what it was like, that's what was going on inside my head, I couldn't control it, I couldn't stop it and I couldn't change it. That done fuck all for my mood, infact I'd go as far as to say it put me back so much. See that was the other problem, I should never have been on social media with my mindset, I was of a very, VERY fragile mindset, now social media at the best of times is a mindfuck, never mind when you're battling depression and suicidal thoughts. I should have come off of it and ignored it, I didn't and I ended up fucking my mind up just that little bit more.

Most commonly thought words from September -
December

- Useless
- Needy
- Suicide
- Mindset
- Mindfuck
- Trying
- Heavy
- Not today

A lot of that was hard for me to take. Depression is a
pattern that's very hard to break. What is it like, it's like
being in a moshpit, the other side is where you need to
get to and to get there you've got to get through
everyone there. They're the barrier and you've got to try
and push through them. A lot of the time I couldn't even
take a step, I thought about it and then went back to
bed, this went on for months, I would actually lose track
of days because every day just rolled into one another.
(This is getting hard again) I kept getting up and I kept
having my breakfast, hoping that one day I would have
a sort of 'Eureka!' type moment, regreattably it didn't
happen. It was hard going though, I know to a lot of
people being off work because of 'depression' would
seem like a sort of free pass to just... lounge about but
it really wasn't. Every night I'd go to my bed so tired
because all I would do all day is think, I got so fucking
tired of thinking, I mean I really did because it was all I
would do, god I got so fucking bored of it. Why was I
thinking? Thinking never resolved anything because all I
would fucking think about was my fucking past. Nothing
good came from that, I would take my anti-depressant,

have my breakfast and then go back to sleep. I would think, I would think, I would think.... (I got soooo tired of thinking, everything was just mush, everything got clumped together and would manifest itself as this big cycle, it would NEVER stop, it never gave me peace, I couldn't even lie in the bath without thinking, it never, ever stopped.......) By the end of it and when I was sitting with the pills in my hand I had thought myself quite literally to death, by the time I got there I was actually relieved, I was actually thinking 'Thank fuck, now I won't have to think anymore', that's what that done to me, over four months it had eroded everything inside me to dust and all I could think about was death, I mean what the fuck, I control my mind, my mind doesn't control me, I mean surely that's the way it should be right?

Wrong. That for me was the battle right there, that key thought was the difference between my winning and losing. I fucking knew that if I could control my mind, I would win and if it controlled me, I lost, up until December my mind definitely controlled me and that's why I actually lost, just because I'm still here doesn't mean I won. I suffered a painful defeat and if it wasn't for my brother reacting and phoning 999 I wouldn't be here, I would have died. So yes, I did suffer a defeat but in the minutes, hours and days to follow after that I started to focus on beating this again. Was it easy to do so? No, absolutely not but trying to take my life and failing gave me a reason to start trying to defeat it again. I'd been to that place and I dared to set my feet over the edge, I made peace with myself and decided that life was for me again, this was it, I was going to give this my all and try to be the type of person I knew

I could be. The type of person I had always dreamed about being but had never had the balls to actually be.

So I tried to return to work one week after attempting suicide. My work quite rightly turned me away, regardless of how positive I felt there was no way I was ready to return, the thought was there and my intentions were good but no way was that my next move, I'm grateful to my employer throughout this whole time, they were amazing. Once again, another example of me being surrounded by excellent people. My support network is amazing. Unfortunately both myself and my employer both decided that we should part company, it was however the right thing to do as we both agreed that I needed to take some time to focus on my rehabilitation, it was correct and I'm glad that I did take that time, it gave me a period of time to kick-start my recovery and start to build up my mental strength.

Chapter Four: Me, Myself & My Mind

I've never felt as if me and my mind were one entity, I've just always felt that either I've controlled it or more often than not it has controlled me. A lot of the times I think I could have controlled it but I think I've let it slip.

I've never really been one for dealing with drama, some people have way too much it going on in their lives and personally I can just do without it. I'm actually a really simple being. All I really want in life is to have a decent job, a nice house, a games console and a few beers, seriously if I could have that then I will actually be contented. I know a lot of people are focused by money and unfortunately in these times it's hard to come by. I wouldn't say money isn't a priority, it is but it's not my ultimate end game. After everything I've been through and everything I've overcome it's time I got back to basics. I need to start looking at things that make me happy, a few of them include:

- Watching/playing snooker
- Playing xBox/Mega Drive
- Listening to music, going to gigs
- Walking the dog
- Spend time with the family

I mean realistically that's all my heart yearns for, I really don't want a lot out of life. If I had lots of money I'd be dead by the time I was forty. I wouldn't be good with a lot of money, it's a good thing I'm not really talented, if I was in the public eye I'd be an absolute fucking nightmare. I think about a lot of things, for example I hate how the UK has this massive 'celebrity culture', to be honest I couldn't give two fucks who wins Big Brother, who wins X-Factor, what retard 'wins' Geordie Shore and who eats the most bugs in 'I'm A Celebrity', is it news worthy? No. Do I give a fuck? No. I just don't see why we get so bothered about a group of halfwits trying to out ego each other. I shouldn't really read the papers or watch TV, it just has a tendency to get my blood boiling but I digress, it's probably better if I leave that behind or things will get ugly really quickly.

Anyways, moving on. So I've never had difficulty relating to others but I have had difficulty with relating others to me. I tried for some years to let people in and see what I was seeing but I could never manage it. I think in a way that I never really wanted people to get it so I could retain some form of individuality and uniqueness. Now though I just don't see that as the best way to go, I've got a life to live. I've got a life that I tried to throw away five months ago. I want to try to help people that feel the same as me, people who suffer, struggle and have to fight to survive. If that means tearing myself down and re-building myself then so be it. For the first time in my life I've regained full control of my mind and I want to use that strength to help other people. I wouldn't go as far as to say it's my calling, that would be an incredibly pretentious thing to say, I've chosen to no longer hide behind my feelings and I want to share them with people. I have lived way too long in silence and in fear and to be honest I'm not going to stand for it anymore. Whenever I look back to my past I've always had a sense of being ashamed but I don't see why I should be? I mean why should I be ashamed or disappointed at something a lot of us go through? Why have I allowed myself to in some way feel inadequate when really I should be proud of all that I have achieved.

This is exactly the way that I'm going to approach things and this is the way I've been thinking for the last two - three months, I've started to appreciate that the way that I feel isn't unique to me, it's something that a lot of people suffer from and I'm tired of the stigma that surrounds it. Mental health issues are just as important as physical health issues, just because you can't see a problem doesn't make it any less important. I felt very conscious about my problems and only a handful of people really knew what I had to endure. Now I'm not saying I'm going to be shouting things from the rooftops when I'm not well but I'm going to speak to someone about it. Rather than me sitting suffering in silence I'm going to talk about my issues and tackle it head on. A lot of people have that fear and believe me when I tell you it really isn't nice, it's a fucking horrible place to be and I wouldn't wish it on anyone. For the first time in my life I've now got the strength to talk about and tackle any issues that I have. Depression is a taxing illness and if we can talk about it more, we can help to break down the walls that's put up.

That being said though I know it's not easy. I went for hours, even days at a time in a state of numbness. I didn't want to go out, I didn't want to stay in. I wanted to be with my family, I wanted to be on my own. I could never settle, I didn't sleep well, I didn't eat well and I didn't really take care of myself. Once again though it wasn't through lack of effort, it was just some days were hard. The strangest thing was though although I neglected myself the house was kept spotless. I done the washing when it needed done, I always made sure that dusting, hovering, bleaching was done. I tidied the livingroom, changed my bedding and made sure everything was clean, so I could look after the house but then I struggled to maintain myself. I think more often than not it was out of sheer boredom, I had the worst thing that someone of my mindset could have... a lot of time. I wasn't really seeing anyone so I had lots of time to myself and that was hard.

There were times I was close to crying, there were days where I would sit on the couch and just look out the window, I wouldn't really do anything else, I'd just... sit. I wouldn't eat for hours, there were days I didn't eat. There was a time where I wore the same pyjamas for five days, I didn't have a bath, I didn't do anything. I just sat there, I sat there and I just... looked out of the window. That's all I done, it was all my mind would allow me to do and I could do absolutely nothing about it. I was helpless, trapped in my own head. There were no physical limitations, there was nothing to actually stop me from doing something but my mind would NOT allow me to do anything. As I'm getting into this I'm beginning to understand myself just what I'm saying, as I'm looking back it wasn't a state of mind. I was imprisoned within my mind, the tablets didn't do anything so I was basically trapped. Now you take that over a period of months, not just one or two days, this was every day I had to fight this off, I had to summon strength day after day to fight this, I fought so hard for so long and in the end I gave up.

I can't sit here and say this'll never happen again, I wouldn't be so foolish or so arrogant to say that. What I need to do daily is to control what goes on inside of my head. That alone won't keep the demons out but it gives me a better chance of managing them, I don't think this is something that I'm ever going to defeat, it's something that I will always need to keep an eye on though. I know when things aren't right, I know what the warning signs are and from now on I'm damn sure if I see any of them they'll be heeded. It's like I'm being told 'you're not feeling right', what happens is:

- A few days before I'll be completely hyperactive
- Then I'll want to 'have a few drinks'
- Then I'll start drinking excessively
- Then I'll start listening to softer music i.e. Kelly Clarkson, Mazzy Star
- Then I'll feel like shit and not want to talk to anyone.

Normally I heed these warning signs and have a few days to myself, the problem was in my last job no-one knew I struggled with depression. Now I put this 100% on myself as I never said to anyone this was the case, when I started to have my struggles listed above I ignored them and carried on as normal and this links back to what I was saying about stigma. I was so scared to mention that I had mental health issues that I made myself really bad before I spoke up. I got to a point where I could no longer cope and I got myself in all sorts of trouble. I never ever want to go through that again, if I had just spoken to someone at the start when I began to feel bad then it could have quite easily meant I could have managed my situation better. I would urge anyone reading this if you don't feel right then talk to someone. Please talk to someone, anyone. Me not talking to someone very nearly cost me my life, I came perilously close, way too close. Now what I've said above may look like I'm blaming myself, I'm not. I'm saying I was scared to talk to someone about what was going inside of me, a mistake that I'll never make again.

There's a lot going on inside me most of the time, I'm not very good at relaxing or doing nothing. I've always got to be doing something which I don't think helps. One thing I'm definitely looking at doing this year is relaxing more. So things like taking more baths, playing more snooker and get out more with the dog. I think that's something I have definitely neglected over the years and it definitely doesn't do me any favours, over the last few months I've been getting better at it and now that I've started work I've put in some groundwork into a work/life balance. I think that's going to be really important for the months and years ahead. Before my problem was that I would always take my work day home with me and vice versa, I never had clear boundaries and I suffered for it. Now I'm not saying I'm going to get this right 100% of the time but if I can get it working for me this will help with me keeping control of my mind and as I've stated earlier, this is really important for me. I don't know why I've never really been able to relax, it's just something that I've always sucked at, I'm always 'on tilt' it seems, like always on edge, tight, rigid. Once again things that do not help when trying to stay in control of my emotions.

My life isn't easy, now I'm not saying that so I can illicit tonnes of sympathy or get a big hug but it's really not easy. I feel passionately about a lot of things and they seem to hit me harder than what they hit the average person. For example I can't read or watch anything to do with animal cruelty, that just reduces me to tears instantly. I feel as if somehow my perception to things like that has a heightened level of sensitivity, it reduces me to rubble on the spot, especially if it contains anything to do with dogs, I love dogs unconditionally and any sort of cruelty towards them makes me want to find the perpetrator and rip their testicles out through their mouth. I apologise for the super graphic nature of that but I feel very very strongly about matters like that. You really don't want to get me started on what I would do to people found guilty of animal cruelty. I'd make Jack Bauer look like a pussy.

With that in mind I'll move on. So you'll remember I said I've never felt that me and my mind were one single entity, I do genuinely feel that they are two separate components and my fight is going to be to get them working as one, I've never really felt that we work together, I always feel that me and my mind are fractured, I feel there's something that doesn't quite match up. Like I always feel that we're at odds and I'm always fighting for control. Maybe I over-think it too much, maybe I don't think about it enough? I actually don't know to be honest, it's a struggle and it's a pretty big drain on my mental resources, it takes up so much of my time and it's tiring. It affects my day-to-day workings, it affects my social interaction, it limits what I can and can't do and most importantly and critically of all it plagues my sleep. When I'm not in control of my mind I don't sleep, I just.. don't. it doesn't matter what I do I just will not fall asleep until about 3am and if I'm up at 6am then I don't need to paint you a picture of what the next day is like. This is why I'm hammering home the point of me being control of my mind, not my mind being in control of me. If I can keep doing what I'm doing and I'm in control I can shape my own future. I'm working so hard to be all I can be and it's imperative that I completely manage my emotions and continue to keep on top of things, I've worked too hard to make it to thirty-three years old, I need to hammer this home.

So what have I been doing, well:

- I'm not worrying as much
- I'm not drinking as much
- I'm not over-thinking as much
- I've been relaxing more
- I'm learning to be comfortable in my own skin
- I'm getting better at switching off.

All of those things combined make a massive difference, if I don't worry I don't stress, when I don't stress I don't drink, when I don't drink I relax more and when I relax more I tend to find I sleep better. Now that may sound like I'm stating the fucking obvious, I'm not, the way I look at it is all these small things combined equate to a huge difference in the way my life works. Each of those statements above are small parts which are part of a plan I put in place nearly six months ago, it's taken a lot of time and effort but it's something that was necessary to stop myself suffering. I'm not saying that for the rest of my life if I work to these principles I'll never suffer from depression but in terms of managing my thoughts and the cycles depression brings this has definitely been a keeper. I used to be really self-conscious, like I got up in the morning and I would scrutinise everything, I hated how I looked in the mirror, I didn't like my face and I could never find anything to wear. Now bear in mind this was all before I'd even left the fucking house so automatically I was behind, because I got up, lumbered to the bathroom, picked faults in everything I could see I was already behind, I had already said to myself 'I'm a loser', 'I suck', I had basically admitted defeat before my day had begun. I hated it but I couldn't stop it, I tried to see the positives but I just couldn't.

Well, fuck that. I do not want to live the rest of my life like that, I'll be damned if I'm going to live the rest of my days with a frown on my face and wallowing in self-doubt. That is no existence for me, yea' there's some days I'll get up and I don't look my best but I take that on the chin and just get on with it. 99.9% of days I get up, shave my head with a razor, take a good look in the mirror and I know that I am going to boss the day. I want to start like a winner. Because then if I start like a winner I stride on my walk to the train station, I walk confidently into work and then I'm already ahead of the game. It's about the mindset, I'm working on a permanent change of my mindset, it might take me six months, it might take me sixty years, all I know though is if I focus on the positives rather than my negatives I'll have a better chance of beating this and living a fulfilling and meaningful life, that's the plan anyways, whether it works out like that time will undoubtedly tell.

When I look at the person I was back in December and the person that I am now it's like night and day, I'm so much more confident now and although I'm looking forward I find it rewarding to just take a glance back to the person that I was. Six months ago I was a shell of my former self, I looked ill, I was ill. I hid behind a pair of yellow sunglasses I didn't want other people looking at me, I wanted to feel invisible, human contact and interaction scared the hell out of me. The only time I would actually feel comfortable is when I spoke to my doctor every Wednesday, I genuinely looked forward to that as it meant I had gone another week without suicide, I'd made it another week and I had fought hard another week. Aside from that I never really felt comfortable being around anyone, my parents, my friends and even my brother who I shared a house with. I didn't feel as if I was worth anything, I felt miserable, poisioned, I felt as if I was insignificant, low, I felt as if I was nothing. I didn't feel as if I was worthy of anyone else's time, my conversation was a waste of my breath and I was a waste of their time. When I talked to professionals it felt as if I was making it up, I was being melodramatic and a hypochondriac, I genuinely felt that I myself was worth absolutely fucking nothing, it was a period of my life where I would quite happily have upped sticks, left and not said a fucking word to anyone. It was horrific.

Chapter Five: Self-Depreciation & Appreciation

I don't class myself as a good person, I have a niece and a nephew that I never see, it's not that I don't want to see them it's just I don't see myself as a positive influence as an uncle, plus my fear of children doesn't help my cause either... Seriously I have a huge fear of children, the farther I'm away from them the better, they give me the utter fear. Remember Rodney (Nicholas Lyndhurst) from Only Fools & Horses and his fear of Damien? Yea', that pretty much encapsulates me. There are three things that I am utterly terrified of, in no specific order they are:

- Children

- Wasps
- Spiders

These are three things that give me the utter and absolute fear, there are probably one hundred things I would do before I ever had to be near any of the above. I just hope that my niece, nephew, (big) brother and wife understand I don't take any part in their life because I'm scared of children, I don't feel I have anything in common with them and my obvious battles mentally. I don't know if that makes me a bad person, I just hope that they understand that there are reasons for my absence.

So at the moment I stay with my folks, I did stay in a really nice flat but due to my (little) brother moving in with his girlfriend in January and my work situation I had no choice but to move back in with the folks, it's fine, I love my parents but I don't like the person that I am when I'm here. My mood is very changeable and I don't like not being able to help/contribute with washing/ironing/tidying etc. My Mum has those covered but then again she always has done. I really don't like the person that I am and I feel that my folks are far too nice to me. I am looking to get my own place in Glasgow but this'll be after a few months when I've had time to bed myself into this job. At the age of thirty-three I just keep thinking that I should be doing better. I have very high-standards for myself, I always have done and I think that I always will do. It's just the way I am, I have an extraordinary high drive and I know no other way. I want to achieve in life, in that respect I class myself like other people.

I take my life very seriously, now that's not an obvious statement as much as it looks like one. I think a lot about where I want to be in five years, I think about my career, I think about what's going to happen when my parents eventually go, I think about a lot, it may not look it at times but I'm very good at looking like I'm thinking of nothing when infact I'm thinking about everything. I always think about everything, it's a blessing and a curse in equal measures, some days I use it to plan ahead and sometimes I think myself to death with 'what if's' and 'buts', it depends on what mindset I'm in, some days it's really hard going, this is why I'm trying to just slow things down a little bit, my mind tends to race and I can get carried away. That needs to stop.

Also, I don't know if it's such a good thing that I manage to be able to think really deeply when I don't look as if I am, it runs along similar lines to my ability to be able to hide how I'm really feeling, let's be honest that didn't really work out too well last time when I was with my previous employer so maybe I should look at dropping that. I think I should treat a 'not so good day' exactly as that, then at least I'll know I'm not forcing smiles or making myself worse. Does that make sense? To me it does but I don't know if it does to you. I'm trying here! So going back to my niece and my nephew, I think I'm doing the right thing but it doesn't feel as if I am? Now that statement isn't deliberate, it's an example of many things in my head where I think one thing but I feel another, I think it would be best for all concerned if I stay out of their lives and as I eluded to earlier it's not a selfish thing, I want to see them grow up and make successes of their selves, I just don't think that me being in their lives is going to be good for me or them, I may be wrong but I don't think I am. For once I'm going to trust my gut and go with the thing that feels right. I just hope one day they understand my reasoning and my logic behind this decision.

Although I try I find it very hard to like the person that I am, I look at other people and I wish I was them, I look at smart people, funny people, people that can dance, people that invent things, people that seem to just find a way to get through life. I'm quite envious of other people, I wouldn't go as far to say jealous because I'm really not the jealous type. I just can't seem to settle on the person that I am, I've tried different looks, tried having a beard and being clean shaven, I really have trouble being myself, I can't settle on something that I'm happy with, my appearance is really important to me because if I'm not happy with how I look there's a good chance that I won't be happy with myself. If I'm not happy with myself then I'm not going to be happy mentally and if I'm not happy mentally then… well, you kind of know how that is going to pan out, for myself it really is not going to go well. I've been there and it's not a pretty place to be.

Do you know what I sometimes do? I don't know if I should even share this but I'm going to anyway, I sometimes imagine that one of my friends has access to my mind, it happens sometimes when I'm in work, sometimes when I'm playing snooker, it happens even when I'm just lying in bed. I imagine they've got access to my mind, like when someone from IT takes control of your computer and they can see what you see? That's what I imagine, I think how I normally think but only someone else has eyes and they can see exactly what I'm thinking. That's quite weird eh? I don't know what triggers it, I've tried so hard to work it out but I've just not been able to work out quite why I think that. The thing is that it seems to re-focus me, it tends to weed out the bad thoughts and channel the good but as you'd expect that's only a temporary state, it never lasts longer than ten to fifteen minutes, fuck knows how that started, I don't know if I believe it or not but I think the reason that I do it is to try to let people in, even if it's not real it's almost like I'm trying to open myself up. Strange.

Another thing that I do which I don't like is I tried to get everyone to like me, well I done that up until I started my new job and I couldn't stop it. I really did not like that about myself at all, why was I trying so hard? I wasn't in high school, I didn't need to be popular, fuck sake in high school I didn't even try to get people to like me so why was I doing it as an adult? It's totally mystifying but thankfully I don't do that now. I'd much rather people didn't like me for the person that I actually am rather than them like me for the person that I'm not. Now that I do understand because it's almost became like a mini-mantra that I practise, I think it's a good one as well because I'd rather be natural than to pretend to like someone or fake laugh at a joke that I just don't find funny. Seriously I'm thirty-three, I need to stop acting like I'm thirteen when it comes to new surroundings and new beginnings.

So, that is definitely enough of the negatives, I know I said earlier that I didn't think I'm a good guy but I really am. I mean I am one of the good guys and that's one of the reasons I've got so many great people around me. I attract people to me and I think I just have something that is natural to me, now I know I said something different earlier but I have to have something, I don't have the kind of friends that I have if I'm an arsehole. I treat people how I like to be treated, I listen, I'm attentive and I'm a fucking good laugh on a night out. I also have a tremendous/inhuman amount of patience, I'm not even kidding I have tolerance and patience above human limits, I don't know how but I just do, it's just my luck I have 'superpowers' that would make me the worst superhero ever. I mean you have Superman, Batman and then you have me, 'Super Patience... Man', I bet I'd have one of those costumes where I'd have a cardboard plate with holes cut out so I could see, stupid cheap green tights and the classic white pants over them. I mean what would my purpose even be?

(In heroic voice) I am Patience Man, I am here to rid the world of mis-understanding and...

Oh fuck that, even I'm fucking bored of that and I've only just thought of it. So yea' I wouldn't be a great superhero but I do actually and genuinely have an inhuman amount of patience and tolerance, it serves me well. One of the main reasons that I've been able to build up my strength is because I've been focusing a lot more on my positives rather than my negatives. Although I don't have my own place just now I still find reasons to look forward. I need to look forward, now I don't like that word, 'need' but it's true, I do actually **need** to start looking forward, the time is right for me to start looking to the future, I have spent the majority of my life looking back and to be honest I'm absolutely fucking sick of it, has it got me anything? No. Has it been healthy for me? No. Has anyone ever achieved anything whilst constantly obsessing and focusing on the past? Absolutely fucking not. So why have I been so focused on it, what has me pointing a laser beam at my past and constantly bringing it up actually proven? It's proven absolutely fuck all. I don't want to be seventy and looking back thinking 'what if':

- What if I just embraced life instead of worrying?
- What if I accepted my past is my past and can't be changed?
- What if I had lived a little

I don't want to be *that* guy. I don't want to live a life with regret, fuck me I've got more regrets than I care to count. I don't need another thirty/forty years of them. Fuck that, I **won't** allow that to happen, I've been building my strength up over the last six months and the time is right for me to not only take control but to start living my life, I don't want to live in fear any more. I won't.

Another problem I have is that I never know what I want and I never seem to settle in one place for long, when I'm in the house I want to go out, when I'm out I want to go home, when I'm in work I want to be outside, I just don't know what I want to be it. I'm constantly wishing time away and I don't like it. I think a lot to myself that I should be living in the now, living in the present because there's going to come a day when I don't have the luxury of time. Once again and it's a recurring theme throughout this but it's about mindset, I'm the one that controls my emotions, I'm the one responsible for managing myself daily so ultimately it's up to me. I know I'm making this sound super simple and I know it's not but you get the jist.

I still really don't like myself, not as much as I should, I still think that I've got a lot I need to address before I would be content within myself, although I've made a lot of progress I wouldn't say I'm happy. I wouldn't say that I'm unhappy but I'm not content, I'm not satisfied, I still drive myself nuts sometimes with my thought processes, I still wander and lose control of my thoughts, I'm absolutely fucking terrible at concentrating, I can concentrate for so long and then I just switch off, I start daydreaming and wandering away to what I done at the weekend, what am I doing tonight, I look at people and I often ask myself what's going on in their head, what are they thinking, what's stressing them, what makes them tick. I spend a lot of time thinking and imagining what other people are going through, I can't stop it. When I'm on the train I like a lot of others participate in the sport of 'people-watching', I'm intrigued by people's individual mannerisms, from the way they sit down to the way they communicate with one another, it's just something that interests me, once again I don't know why.

It's not easy to change engrained thought processes and it's certainly not easy when you're not happy within you.

Is this an admission that I'm not 100% happy with myself at the moment? From what I've started writing in the previous paragraph I would have to say yes, yes it is. That right there is a fight I think I'm just always going to have, I'd love to sit here and say that I am completely happy and completely contented but the truth is, I'm not. When I was eighteen I started writing and when I say writing I mean poems and things, not writing as I am now. Over the space of ten years I had well over one thousand things written down and the majority seemed to focus on one thing, how unhappy I was. A lot of my writings hammered home the fact that I was deeply unhappy, at one point in 2007 I had actually written a sort of suicide note saying goodbye to everyone, the writings in that were very concise, honest and to the point. I guess if you're writing something like that you really have to be honest. Unfortunately I scrapped all of my writings after I nearly committed suicide in 2011, I felt that if I didn't have the writings then I wouldn't refer back to my past, the logic was there but I'm not sure it really made any difference. I'd love to say it did but here we are four years later and being honest I still have similar struggles to what I have them. I mean the stuff that I'd written wasn't clever, it was just basic rhyming so for example I'd write something like:

'These days they just get longer, my head just isn't changing

I'm tired of putting on this front, this happiness I'm feigning

I wish that I was better, I wish I wasn't such a stranger

My strength is slowly waning, I think my life's in danger'.

I mean it's not brilliant but it had a simple structure to it, it did also help because it forced me to think about what was actually going on inside of me. I don't know, do I really want to start digging this up again? I'm not sure I'm ready for it but then this links back to not knowing what I want, it's like The Clash with 'Should I Stay Or Should I Go', I don't fucking know and it really pisses me off, I don't think I should think this much, in many ways I'd love to just be an airhead, just having the wind whistle between my ears, not think of anything and just live a life. I mean really that sounds brilliant instead of my head, I hate the fact I can't switch off and I really mean that.

When I said this was going to hurt right at the start I knew there was going to be a point where it was going to start really hurting, I'm at this point because what I'm basically saying is that I am not happy with myself, I kind of thought that I wasn't but this has confirmed it. I mean maybe this is what my life is going to be about. Maybe I'm just always going to be on the edge, stuck in the middle of happiness and struggle, maybe that's my place, maybe that's where I'm going to have to fight my battle from every day. Yea' actually this is really beginning to hurt, I feel like I'm pressing really hard with a salt covered finger into what I thought was a healed wound. It's not a healed wound, it's still open and it still feels raw, I wasn't prepared for this, I thought I was passed this, I guess I wasn't, I'm not ready and it may not be a bad thing, this brings me nicely onto my next major struggle...

Alcohol…

Oh god this is a bad one, I have a really tempestuous relationship with alcohol, it's been the cause of so much of my problems and it's something I've got to constantly fight against. I can abuse alcohol quite easily and it only happens over the course of a couple of days, see that's another weight on my mind and yet something else that needs managed. It's fucking hard work because I know once I get started on alcohol I don't stop. It starts with a couple of pints and within a couple of days it can spread to having six cans a night, not just a week, a **night.**

I like to have a couple of pints on my own, I actually do. As much as I like going out with people and having a laugh I do have to constantly find the balance between being around people and being on my own. Yet another thing that I've got to find a balance on, as this goes on I really want you to see just how much I balance daily, no wonder I have 'not so good days', due to the strength I've got that enables me to keep them from turning into bad days, bad days are just… death, those are the days where I just want to run away from everyone and dive under my duvet. I want to shut the world out, turn my phone off and just ignore everyone. **These are the days where I DO NOT AND I WILL NOT TOUCH ALCOHOL.**

If I touch alcohol then I'd be as well just doing it, I done it once and I will never ever do it again. It was four years ago and I still remember it. I remember walking around Glasgow bawling my eyes out, I still remember posting a last picture on Facebook, I remember the clothes that I was wearing and I still remember every single detail of that day. Alcohol and bad days are the absolute recipe for my own personal disaster. I will never ever do that again.

But going back to alcohol, I've got an example of just how dangerous a relationship I have with it. I finished training on Friday (22/05/2015) and went out bevvying with my training group, they're a great bunch of guys and I'd been looking forward to it all week. I went out at about 13:30 and I left at approximately 19:30, I lifted the wrong laptop bag as well, fanny. Now I'd had a good day, I didn't have any sort of clouds over me and I was in a good place. For absolutely no reason at all I started crying whilst walking down Sauchiehall Street, now I don't know what caused this, all I know is there were similarities to **THAT** day in 2011, not quite to the same extent but the tears were real and I felt miserable. Now that was on a day where I felt great and I'd had a great day, things can change that fast in my head so it's absolutely critical that I keep a really close eye on things. As I said, things in my head can turn not at the drop of a hat but pretty fucking quickly. Thankfully my bestie was on hand to come pick me up and make sure I was ok.

It just goes to show you even when you think that everything is ok you've got to be really careful. Actually I'll rephrase that because that's not right. It just goes to show when I think everything is ok I've got to be really careful. I don't think I was particularly drunk, I reached my limit and for once I decided to go instead of trying to blitz my way through it. I don't know what happened although I have a theory. I've just started this job, (I may have mentioned this) I've kept my cards pretty close to my chest and on Friday I was passing my book around, the one I wrote six months ago. Now my theory is this, even though I didn't look inside this book, even though I didn't read the contents did they embed in my head and as my alcohol consumption increased did the thoughts amplify subliminally? Did they somehow get past me when I was busy getting merry? It may not be definitive but it's definitely plausible. Something must have happened because I went from happy to crying in the space of a seven minute walk. The mind truly boggles, well.. mines does anyway.

Maybe it would be better if I gave up alcohol? I mean looking at all I've been through it's been a constant throughout it. I don't know if it's been the actual root cause but it's played a significant part in my mental capitulations over the years. Maybe I just need to get a better handle on it, fuck off who am I kidding I depend on alcohol too much to give it up. I'm not even going to try to kid myself that I'll give it up because I just won't. I mean really Davy, don't kid yourself or anyone else. You'll notice a key word there when I was mentioning alcohol. I didn't say I 'enjoy alcohol' too much, I said 'I depend on alcohol too much' and that is exactly what it is, it's a dependency and one of the reasons I'm glad I don't have thousands of disposable income is I would blow it on alcohol. (Remember what I said when I left 3? Exactly) So I need to control my dependency because like my happiness it's all about balance. Ugh I make my own head hurt at times, I've just read the last two paragraphs back and it just confirms my relationship with alcohol, it's fucked up. I don't know, maybe I should actually look at it more and decide if I really want to pursue it. I mean, I gave up sex pretty easily, surely alcohol should be an easier thing to give up? Or am I looking at that in too much of a simple manner? I can never decide if I'm looking at something too simply or too complex. Yet another reason as to why my mind blows a fuse every now and then.

I'm not sure I want to continue on to be honest, since I've been writing I've noticed a change in my mood, I can feel it, I don't know if it's because I'm actually seeing what I've been thinking or if I'm digging deeper than I thought, when I first started this I thought this was going to just be a recap/building block of what I've done over the last six months, as it's turned out that's just not the case at all. This is getting deeper and I think it's going to get a lot more brutal, I can feel it. There's something deep down there, I can feel it's presence at the back of my mind. Oh well, better try and find it then eh?

Point of reference, at the time of writing this it's 18:45 on 25/05/2015, I've just settled down with a couple of beers. I did say that I would inform you when alcohol was involved. It seems only fair that I keep my promise. So the last few days have been very strange. I wouldn't say I don't feel right, I'd say I feel ok, just not... right. Like I feel ok but I feel something, I can feel something that's burning away, almost like something faintly drilling at the back of my mind, trying to bore it's way to the front. Maybe this whole 'tearing myself down and re-building' me idea wasn't so good after all. I think a better way to word it because of the way I'm feeling is I am un-hinging myself and then trying to re-hinge myself, that's how I feel at this exact moment. I'm not going to lie I don't really feel anything at the minute, I just feel...

I don't know what I feel, I'm having trouble really telling you how I feel, I'm trying to work it out but there's just nothing there. I mean I feel good about going back to work tomorrow, that's a start. I'm looking forward to seeing the guys, I've had three days off and they've been ok. I mean apart from crying on Friday night after leaving the pub yea' it's been a good one. I mean it has been ok, I think maybe I drank too much and was thinking about the book? I mean this was the first time I've been in public and discussed it since I wrote it. Also alcohol was involved so maybe that's what caused it? I'm still trying to decipher that one, I keep playing it over and over in my head and to be honest I'm still no further forward with it. The problem is that I can't leave it alone, I've got to just nit-pick it and analyse it, I've got to look for a point, I feel like a really bad version of Columbo, like a REALLY bad version. I'm no further forward so I'm going to try and leave it. I mean it's happened, it's in the past, I can't change it. I mean.... that's where it needs to stay.

takes a sip

I think I'm making things too complex again, I'm burning through mental resources un-necessarily and looking for things that really don't matter. I mean why am I trying to run over events with a fine tooth-comb when I don't really need to. All that I am really doing is using up energy that could be better saved for when I really need it like a not so good day or worst-case scenario a bad day. That's really been a theme of today, I've not really been thinking a lot but I feel tired mentally, I mean that may have something to do with the fact I'm writing all of this but I don't think it is. Even though I've literally just said I'm using up un-necessary energy and I need to save it I'm still using it.

'I'm still thinking and pondering, I'm sitting and wondering,

I'm waiting and watching, for the thoughts that are walking

Why won't this go and leave me alone,

I want to stop thinking, and be on my own.'

Ugh I'm getting annoyed with myself now. I hate my mind. No doubt it hates me too.

Chapter Six: Nothing in Particular

I fantasise a lot, I often come up with scenarios that are never ever going to play out in my head. I hate them but I can't stop seeing them. One that really pisses me off is when I wake up in the morning. I go through my morning routine, I get up, wash my face, shave my head and then have breakfast. Then for no plausible reason I fantasise about taking a penalty kick and doing a backflip in front of a cheering crowd. I mean...

What the fuck? What is that? That makes no fucking sense whatsoever.. What am I even thinking, that's never going to happen. But most mornings it comes into my head, eventually I forget it and get on with my day. See stuff like that really screws with me because I'm not analysing everything but my brain comes up with this really stupid fantasy. I've got another one. When I listen to a particular group of songs I imagine it's me singing it on karaoke and I reduce people to tears, I MEAN WHHAATTTTT! Oh fuck off Davy what the fuck is that, that also makes no sense, the songs I do this to are:

'Umbrella' by 'Rihanna'

'Gone Away' by 'The Offspring'

'My Heart Is A Fist' by Papa Roach

I don't play these songs now because I'm so tired of playing out that 'fantasy', see that's the type of shit that's going on inside my head, that's not normal, I can't convince myself it's normal. Do you know what I've started doing to try and block these stupid things out? I've started focusing on an imaginary pink ball at the front of my head, not only does it divert your focus away from stupid thoughts and fantasies but it also comes in handy for making yourself look blank. It comes in handy on the commute to work, I HATE business conversations at 7:47 in the morning. Seriously mate, shut the fuck up or I'll beat you to death with your own laptop. I need a huge mug of coffee before I can do anything in the morning. Listening to conversations about spreadsheets, projections and calendar appointments before I've had coffee is a very dangerous game to play. You are taking your life in your hands when you do that. Another thing that annoys me on the train is people that have full blown meetings over the phone before 8am.. Seriously mate/hen get a life. It can wait until you get into Glasgow, trust me it's not going to go away. I swear a lot of them are on the phone to their voicemail or something trying to look important, I have my doubts about people having these conversations THAT early in the morning. I think I'm just not a morning person, I'll rephrase that, I am fucking not a morning person, I generally come to around 12pm, that's when I start being productive, either that or after my third coffee.

I've never really been one for small talk, I can be quite fidgety, I don't really have any confidence in my small talking skills at all unless I'm in the pub in which case I never fucking shut up. I do prefer myself on a night out, I'm a much more entertaining guy after I've had a few beers on a Friday! In general though I'm just not good at small talk, I try but I'm much more comfortable just sitting listening to people rather than getting involved. I always think whatever I've done is boring but then a lot of that links back into how I'm envious of other people. Nine times out of ten I have a perfectly valid weekend, I either go and practice snooker or I veg and play xBox, sometimes I meet my bestie and we hang out for a bit. Some weekends I'm actually quite productive and sit down and do budgets for the month ahead. Ok, that falls into the one out of ten category, I'm not going to try to kid anyone, that is boring as fuck. I don't know what it is but I just can't seem to maintain my confidence, I suck at eye contact as well, I always look away, I think it's to do with the fact that there can be such a thing as too much eye contact? Like someone totally staring through you, yea' I don't wanna be that guy, no-one wants to be that guy. So I've been doing a lot of thinking over the last couple of days and there's one thing I'm going to do on Thursday (Payday! Yey!) and that's buy a pair of big baggy trousers with chains on them, they make me really happy and I would say I've sort of lost my identity a bit without them, I dress nicely now but I don't want that all the time. I want to cut about with them on, have my music turned up and just be that little bit different. I know for a fact that's just not helped me confidence wise, I'm at my best when I look different, I definitely don't feel at my best when I 'look nice'. I mean it's ok, I always present myself nicely enough but I'm not like anyone else, I want that little bit of individuality again, it's a nice feeling to not feel like a clone of the person next to you. Actually the more I start thinking about this the more I want to think about piercings and tattoos. I'd love some new piercings and tattoos, that could be a plan but Thursday is a little bit of time away so I'll wait and see, definitely buying the baggy jeans though, those things are the fucking mutts nuts! Now that's interesting, just typing that I'm going to buy a pair of baggy jeans after payday has perked me up a little bit. I'm actually quite looking forward to that because they do actually make me happy. They're not for everyone I agree but each person has their own thing that makes them happy. For me it's definitely simple, baggy jeans, a t-shirt with a band slogan on it and a pint in one of my two favourite pubs in Glasgow, Rufus T Firefly or the Solid Rock Café, both pubs I frequent and I love them, mainly just because of the awesome tuneage that's played in both establishments. I've spent many a night there with friends. If you've never been I'd highly recommend them!

I need to find some inspiration from somewhere, it gets pretty tiring constantly fighting with yourself, analysing everything you say and do. I need to try to find something that's going to serve me well in life, not something like a mantra but something that allows me to live instead of exist. That for me is a big thing. I don't want to hit sixty, seventy or eighty, looking back and realised that I didn't live my life, I existed it. That for me is not how I want to leave my legacy, I want to leave behind a lifetime of great memories and this is why personally my battle with depression is something I've chosen to write about. I've tried different ways of dealing with it in the past and none of them have worked if I'm being honest. I've tried therapy, I've tried talking to friends and I've even had professional help. I'm not saying it didn't help but I thought by this point I would feel better than what I do. Ugh that sounds like I'm being ungrateful, I don't mean it to sound like that, I'm grateful that so many people have invested so much of their time in me, I just can't shake that feeling that there's something inside of me that's different to everyone else. I think there's a lot I can give to people but I just need to unlock it, there's definitely something yearning inside me, something that says I can do more but quite what that is I don't know. God knows I'm trying to find it, I've spent fifteen years on an emotional rollercoaster and to be honest I think I'm going to be on it for the rest of my life. Maybe I'll never find it, maybe I'll search and search with no luck. Maybe I'll find something, something that I can hold onto and use for the rest of my life. I genuinely don't know, if I did then I wouldn't be sitting here clawing at my mind trying to get in.

There's a point actually, remember what I said at the start about my levels of empathy? It's not just my empathy that's heightened, I feel so much compassion and emotion, I wish I could explain what I feel, I could try but I'd be here for one hundred years, I'll try to give you an insight into the emotion part, it happened two minutes ago so while it's fresh and here's how it broke down. So I was writing the paragraph above when my Dad came in and said he'd managed to find a recording of a TV show that he thought he'd deleted, so I went in, thanked him and watched the end of it. The end scene is magnificent, I don't know if I'm allowed to mention the name of the show so I won't. But the end scene and the accompanying end song that led to credits caused me to go into a stare, the music hit me really hard and I could fill every note, every word and every drumbeat fill my head, it washes over me like a wave, it moves me without trying, it fills my very soul with hope and it makes me forget what I'm worrying about. That's how quickly it happens, certain songs played at just the right time can just make my heart sing, they can just alleviate me from my worries and take me to a place where nothing matters but as I say it's all about timing. I can listen to the one songs one hundred times but unless it's at the exact time that I need it then it's just a song, granted that song might be great but it doesn't give me that freedom, that release. Right now it does and I've not had that for a while. I feel moved, light, floating, I feel as nothing matters, these moments are as important to me as a good nights sleep, with moments like this I can hope again, I feel the freedom of the bars, the crescendo of the vocals, the loving caress of strings and I feel a heart soaring, I feel my heart soaring. I feel good, I feel strong and I write in time with the music. I share a very special bond with certain pieces of music and as of now I'm in time, I'm in tune and nothing can ruin this moment. Just to put into perspective this one moment has the potential to change the course of my next month or so, that's how important these bits of timing are in my life. I absolutely cherish these moments because they don't come around that often, I couldn't even put a number on it because it happens so little. All I know right now I have been carried skyward and I feel like flying. I feel my wings spread and everything lift. It's magical, spiritual and it's happened just when I needed it, when I was beginning to wane a little.

I'm powerless when my mental strength starts to wane, the harder I fight, the worse it gets. I've got to let my not so good days just run because it's better for me. If I try and fight, I make my mental state worse, I know it's coming so I cocoon myself up and wait for it to pass. How could I describe it. It's like another layer appears between me and my mind, it locks me in and doesn't allow me to communicate freely. It walls me up and stops me from being. I've got sit inside my mind for two to three days, let it run and then I'm fine. Now I mentioned earlier about warning signs, I heed them, if any of the warning signs appear then I obey them, they advise me that trouble is coming and I'm glad they do because I get some time to prep, I get some time to ready myself for the coming days, my friends understand, my family understand, my work colleagues understood. This has yet to happen in my new job so when it does I'll have to be brave. It's actually quite a surreal place to be when the not so good days hit. My level of focus just skyrockets, although I can't physically engage in small talk my focus to my work increases ten-fold, it allows me to do what needs to be done but nothing else. I do not question my mind through this time, I'm indebted to it because it's warned me of an impending danger, to this extent me and my mind have an unspoken agreement. He has been so kind to warn me of some unpleasant times on the horizon, I do not speak ill of him and he processes what needs to be processed until I am well again. There are times where me and my mind do work together as a single entity, I like it when we do because we know what needs to be done, I'm thankful to him because he does me a favour, I should maybe be a little more appreciative of my mind. Maybe he'll take this as a thank you, I hope he does. That's the thing though sometimes there is no trigger, sometimes it just.. happens and then I'm left sidestepping and dodging anyone and everyone, sometimes there is just no reason for it. It just engulfs me and I have no choice but to deal with it. I've no choice to accept it and then run with it. These are the days when I'm glad to be on my own, everything makes sense in my head, because of the barrier goes up no thoughts get out, none come in and none cycle, my thoughts don't get into their speed cycle and so I can sleep for a few nights. It's almost like the not so good days are resting me, taking control for a few days and just slowing things down. I'm not going to lie, sometimes I do like these days, they give me time to myself and they give me time to re-energise and re-focus for when the thoughts start their cycle.

That is by far the hardest thing I've got to control, the not so good days are more than manageable but when I can't get a single thought that's when I'm in danger, that's when I need someone around me because I'm stuck, I don't have that protection anymore, my mind has no firewall so the thoughts do as they please, they race out of control and they create a huge internal vortex, I can't settle, I can't focus and I can't sleep, god I fucking hate these days, 'the cycle' doesn't break and it just gets faster and faster, taking every positive thought I've had/I have and just sucking it into the vortex, swallowed whole and not to be seen again. This for me is hell, there is no set routine, there is no kill switch I can engage, whenever I close my eyes all I see are the thoughts, all I see is a hurricane enveloping everything and all. Every single thing I've done wrong in my life comes back at me, taunting and haunting me. Raping me and robbing me, I sit for hours just looking out a window, praying for this to stop, internally pleading with my mind to stop this from happening, our relationship has fractured, I've had no warning so this is all on me. My sleep is broken and deep, my eyes are heavy and bagged. I'm not resting and one day is running into the next without a break. I've had no time to recoup, it's straight into battle and slowly but surely my mental strength starts to suffer as a result. I have to focus so much of my strength on quietening the cycle that it leaves me little else for anything else. I've seen it effect my work, my personal life and before I took my vow of celibacy it even affected that as well. Granted that was a rarity but it still impacted. This for me is the part of my depression that I fear the most, I am so scared of it because I know it's the most susceptible state of mind that I can be in. That's normally when suicidal thoughts start to form and those take a tremendous amount of hard work and controlling. I could tell you just how hard I work at this but I don't think you would ever appreciate just how much effort I've got to put in to stop them. That's not a dig at you, if it comes across as that then god I apologise, I'm trying to convey just what happens at the height/depths of my depression, when I'm at my absolute worst and the tears won't stop flowing, the tears just keep coming and coming. They need to being honest, referring back to how much emotion I feel it's only natural that it erupts at some point, thankfully it happens when I'm in the cycle stage, if I feel it's going to help I'll watch Turner & Hooch, that film guarantees me tears so I put it on and let the tears flow. Am I ashamed to admit this? No. I need to do this because it does help, there is no kill switch, there is no way out. All I can do is sit, barricade myself in and pray that this alleviates, pray that this lifts. Depression is a horrific illness, I mean it just flat out sucks because it can strike at any given point, fortunately the majority of my episodes strike after some warning but when it's cyclic, I'm pretty much fighting it 24/7. Fuck that takes it's toll.

In work it's a horrific discussion to have to have with a manager. I mean it's just not one I'm ever comfortable having. Physically I'm fine, I look ok but if I've got armageddon kicking off in my head then it's best for me to say what's going on. Now I've been fairly lucky in the fact that when it's struck me in work I've had the warning so it's been relatively low-key. I am dreading getting the cyclic depression at work, that would be an absolute horror situation and an absolute fucking nightmare. I'm still scared about opening up to people I'm not comfortable with about my battles, I think that's perfectly natural though, I wouldn't feel comfortable just walking up to someone and blabbering all of what I've written above, I have to manage each person individually. Some people get to see everything that happens and some people only get told at surface level 'I'm not feeling too good today', that's completely deliberate on my part because not everyone needs to know exactly what's happening inside of my head. There is one person that knows everything that goes on inside my head, just one person and my parents don't even know everything. I choose to keep some information from them because this is my battle. I have to fight this and as long as they know I'm either coping or having just one of those days then that's plenty.

I would say if I was to describe my 'depressive personality' I'd definitely say I'm an 'introverted depressive', I like to keep everything to myself and unless I'm specifically asked for info. concerning it then I'll volunteer nothing. I think with the way my mind works it's best I keep things to myself, I delete my Facebook app for a couple of days, I delete any sort of messaging tools that I have and I just wall up until such time I'm ready to emerge again. I used to be the opposite where I shared everything with everyone, that didn't work because not everyone needs to know everything. I have a very close circle of friends that I would trust with anything, if they ask or I need to talk to them they get everything. As I say if I do need to have 'a conversation' with a manager within my new role it's going to be dependent on just what kind of depression I'm suffering from. Hopefully I never have to have the conversation and I can just.. work. That being said though I still think there's a negative stigma surrounding mental health and I don't think it's particularly anyone's fault. It's just.. hard saying to someone 'I don't feel good today' or 'I'm suffering today'. I find it hard, to this day I still find it hard to say to someone because the first thing they do is worry, it's perfectly natural because you're basically saying 'I'm not right' even though nine times out of ten it's temporary.

I'll give you an example. Around the middle of December I made four videos and posted them on YouTube, they ranged from talking about depression to my own struggles with depression to the fact that I felt I was coming out of depression, I think one of them I made when I was drunk.. (cringe..) But I made those videos around the middle of December and less than two weeks later I had been hospitalised once for almost attempting suicide and then again for actually attempting suicide. So when people get worried I completely understand why they do, it must be terrifying for them to know a person is either contemplating or saying they're actually going to do it. I mean that's what I done and I worked my friends and family into a frenzy, I didn't mean to but as I said earlier, I'd had enough, my reasons for living no longer outweighed my reasons for dying, I had ran out of strength, I'd had too many cyclic days and I'd fell into the alcohol trap, my head was fucked and unfortunately I had decided that I'd had enough. I'm not proud of it but I did say that I didn't know if I was going to make it out the other side. I wasn't being dramatic, I was being factual, I didn't know where my battle was going to take me and unfortunately I did give in, I succumbed and I wanted out. I'm not ashamed though, I sit here with my head held high because that battle was personal to me, yea' ok I didn't beat it through sheer willpower but I did eventually beat it and start working towards recovery and re-habilitation. I think it's testament to the sheer amount of mental strength that not only did I beat it but nearly three months to the day that I'd attempted suicide I then applied for, prepped for and then managed to secure the great job that I'm in now. That's what gets me through not so good days, the sheer amount of strength that I have, I managed to come through a horrible period of my life and I didn't just come through it, I also managed to gain employment with a great company and get a great job in Glasgow.

Just on the subject of things not helping me do you not what doesn't help me, when people don't tell me something directly. See if you need to tell me something? Tell me it. Honestly I'm thirty-three years old, I'm pretty sure I can handle it. I mean things like if someone doesn't like me or they have something to say to me. Just come out with it, I hate pussy-footing around, I'd rather just be told something than just sit there and wonder what's going on. Honestly, I'm not going to act like a thirteen year old who's been killed playing Call of Duty, I'm a big boy, I can take whatever is thrown at me, trust me. I've been dealing with this crap for fifteen years, I'm pretty sure I can take anything thrown at me, positive or negative. I just somehow feel as if I get babied, like given watered down versions of things. Trust me, if you've got something to say then please, do me a favour, just give it to me straight. Don't really know where that came from to be honest, just must have been one of those things that has been building up y'know?

So hopefully you'll remember when I said under the right conditions beer allows me to open up just enough? I feel exactly what's been written was exactly what I wanted to get out, over three hours I had two beers and between that and the music from earlier it's allowed me just to cut myself open and bleed a little bit out.

If someone who'd never suffered with depression was to come up and ask me 'What is depression like' I think I would struggle to answer, I mean I know what it's like but could I honestly get across to someone who's never struggled exactly what it's like? Could I encapsulate it? Could I describe it? Do you know something I'm not sure I could without making it sound dramatic. I wouldn't be trying to make it sound like that but I think it would come across as that. How would I describe it, well.. what if I was to say it was like walking into a really strong headwind or trying to push a car up a really steep hill? Would those examples work or would that be too simple an explanation. I mean is the definition of depression constant? No, it's not. I wonder should I maybe use the example I used above that's personal to me and the differences where I have 'warning sign depression' and 'cyclic depression'? Would that maybe be too much? Do you know something I don't actually know if I could describe it. I mean don't get me wrong, I'd give it a fucking good go, there'd be no doubts about that. I guess it would be dependent on the person, one thing I do know about depression is that lots of people suffer from it. I know I mentioned it in my last book but the death of Robin Williams *really* hit me hard. That's what started things off again, that one incident started the cycle again. I was going along ok, ok I was on a bit of a drinking spree but I was managing, then I woke up one morning and heard that Robin Williams had died. Now Robin Williams was in his sixties when he died, I think what that said to me was that I was never ever going to beat depression, I could never outrun it. Up until that point I had convinced myself that I had defeated it. Now when I say I'd defeated it I'm referring to the point in 2011 where I almost attempted suicide. I'd made great strides since then and I was doing well, yea' I still had 'off-days' and 'not so good days' but no real bad days to speak of. That one incident I can pinpoint as where my thinking patterns changed.

I wasn't the same internally, I didn't think the same after that, I started to worry, I started to wonder if this was going to come back again. What would I do if it hit me in my fifties? Who would I have around me? Would I die alone? Would anyone actually care? What if I'm miserable for the rest of my life and I'm constantly trying to outrun the reaper? But... I've beaten depression haven't I? I mean I've came close to suicide but I've not done it, 2011 is past so surely I've nothing to worry about?

WRONG. I started to worry. I started to worry a LOT. I started drinking more, I was having not so good days but ignoring the warning signs that my mind was mapping out for me. I wasn't sleeping. So looking back not only did I ignore my warning sign depression but I also chose to ignore the far more serious cyclic depression. I had started suppressing and that, well wow that worked out well didn't it. I started feeling unwell at the start of August, now when I state I was feeling unwell I am of course referring to my mental state, physically I was ok, just.. ok. The real danger sign came on 16/08/2014 of last year, I started writing poems down again, I wrote a few poems which pointed out quite clearly something wasn't right, once again though rather than facing the problem head-on I ran away from it. So in the months leading up to my breakdown on 01/09/2014 let's look at the timeline of just how things transpired:

- Start to show signs of waning mental strength at the start of August
- Robin Williams dies on 11/08/2014
- **Symptoms of warning sign depression ignored**
- **Signs of cyclic depression ignored**
- Writing about low mood and pain on 16/08/2014
- Drinking heavily from 16/08/2014 until 31/08/2014

So if you look at that you'll see it's a pretty fast decline. Now I'll be the first to admit I crashed through my warning signs and kept going, that was a mistake but that's just how quickly things can change, by the time 31/08/2014 came I was drinking so much that I wasn't even tasting the alcohol, I was drinking to forget, I had drank so much and suppressed so much that by the time I was waiting on the train to work on 01/09/2014 I was broken. I stood at the train station crying. I was thinking about suicide, I was thinking about jumping in front of the train, I was thinking how to say goodbye to everyone, my mind was shot and this was due to the culmination of events I've just described. I mean let's ignore events one, two, four and five and focus on the ones highlighted in bold, I CHOSE to ignore the warning signs, normally my friendly depression I decided to ignore my mind, it told me something wasn't right but instead of heeding, I ignored. Not only that.... Not only that but when I got my far worse friend Mr Cyclic I ignored that as well, to this day I will never understand what was going on in my mind to make me ignore both of these very clear depressive states of mind. I chose to plough on regardless and I basically fucked my mind. The increase in alcohol was massive as well so when you take all of those factors it's not surprising in the space of less than a month I was ruined. That timeline all links together, all of it added together was too much for me to take and by the time I got into work on 01/09 I was a wreck, I couldn't speak, I couldn't speak to my dear friend that sat beside me, god I couldn't even speak to The Samaritans to talk to someone about me wanting to commit suicide, it was that bad I just couldn't talk. My mind was shot and everything was fractured and broken. Everything was just burnt out, my wiring was gone, my links were all fried and by the time it came time to go home I just wanted to sleep.

Now... I'm going to skip ahead here because the next two months were fine, I was well into a course of anti-depressants, something that I'd been strongly against previously. I'd started to rest/recuperate and I started to feel a little better within myself, I didn't really see any of my friends that much though because my state of mind was still paper-thin and I was still highly sensitised to the world around me. Overall though I displayed good strength, I'd avoided alcohol and yea', I felt ok. I done the things that made me happy. I played xBox, I cleaned the house, I maintained the house and I ensured that everything kept ticking over. Now from 03/09/2014 I started seeing my GP weekly, I saw him every week without fail. Throughout this whole experience he is the one person that knows everything that happened, he got the whole timeline and every single rumble and tremor that I experienced. I'd like to thank him for his time and advice. He was an absolute rock and I will never forget all that he done for me. Things started going wrong for me when he said the words 'You can have a few drinks with these tablets', although it didn't happen instantly I began to crave alcohol more and more. I'd put in a lot of effort to ensure that I didn't touch alcohol as I didn't want it interfering with the tablets, I began with one can a week, then I was having a couple of cans a week, then I wasn't taking my tablets some days and then I was having two/three cans every couple of days. Yip unfortunately I was back on the booze and the recovery/recuperation had slowed. Although I never showed any symptoms of cyclic depression I was definitely having a lot of warning sign depression, I did heed it when it came and I pulled my alcohol consumption back but doing things in hindsight I would have definitely stayed off the alcohol. By the time I'd had my brush with suicide and my attempted suicide I was really drinking heavily again. I'm not proud of it and being really blunt in my criticism I was an absolute fucking idiot. You don't get any second chances, once your life is finished then that's it, it's game over, it's done and I never once thought of that. I couldn't think of that, I wasn't in the mindset to think like that.

I.... I deeply and wholeheartedly apologise to everyone that was involved in my life at that time, it must have been an absolutely awful thing to have to deal with, although it wasn't much fun for me it must have been ten times worse for you. I'm sorry, I really am sorry. I **AM SO SO SORRY, I HATE MYSELF FOR EVER PUTTING YOU THROUGH ALL OF THAT. TWO NEAR SUICIDES IN A WEEK EITHER SIDE OF CHRISTMAS. I AM SO.. SO SORRY.**

It's true, I really am sorry for that time but what I'd ask people to bear in mind is that I wasn't me, I was so far away from the person I am it wasn't believable. I felt miserable, I felt vacant, I didn't feel stimulated, I just felt tired, I felt useless, worthless, draining, not worth it, reclusive, distant. I felt as if the world was better off without me, I was better off without me. My family and friends were better off without me. I was a drain on all resources, I wanted the world to empathise with me, I wanted the world with me. I wanted... I wanted people to understand just what hell I was going through. For the first time I was thinking of myself, for the first time I was thinking just about myself. I was thinking about my needs, I was thinking about trying to pull through this but I was failing, my recovery had stopped, my respite had gone, I had used all of my strength and I had ran out. I had exhausted all avenues, I'd used all resources and for the first time, I allowed myself thoughts about dying, I'd softened myself up with six beers and I had decided on 20/12/2014 I was going to be no more, I said goodbye to my friends on Facebook and pulled out a small table from the cupboard.

I stood on it.

I put one foot on the balcony.

I looked down

I looked up,

I looked down

I went to step and then jump, this was it.

At that exact moment the door went with a mighty thud, I stopped. I took myself down and I answered the door. I went with the paramedics and the police and I spent the night in hospital. I felt guilty, I felt sick and I felt horrid that I'd put my friends and family through that. My friends had called the emergency services as they'd got my address details through Facebook.

Less than a week later it happened again only this time I took twenty-one anti-depressants at once, I'd overdosed and text my brother to say goodbye, he phoned an ambulance, I was back in hospital yet again, passing out and vomiting from all the tablets that I'd taken. I spent the night in hospital with my Mum by my side, I kept passing out so I didn't really say much, I was a mess, I just didn't know what to say, what could I say? I'd just attempted suicide. I had given up, I had accepted in my head that I was going to die.

The point I'm trying to make is this. Depression is very much a state of mind, now quite what that state of mind is I can't answer conclusively. I can only speak from experience and my experience is that I get hit in stages. I get some severe and not so severe episodes. It's been five months since all of that happened and things are so much better. I'm staying with my parents until I can get on my feet in my new job and then I'm going to make the move to Glasgow, it's my favourite city and I love the nightlife. I know I'll need to be careful though because there are many pitfalls that I'll need to be wary of, mainly alcohol. I mean I will really need to avoid excessive consumption of alcohol. Things change so quickly in life and in my life I need to do all that I can to ensure I live a full and fulfilling life.

Thank you so much for reading.

Davy

www.ingramcontent.com/pod-product-compliance
Lightning Source LLC
Chambersburg PA
CBHW072309200526

45168CB00014B/1110